V. Kishan

Levodopa and Carbidopa Controlled Release Matrix Tablets

Jagan Mohan Somagoni
Y. Madhusudan Rao
V. Kishan

Levodopa and Carbidopa Controlled Release Matrix Tablets

Formulation and InVitro Evaluation

Lambert Academic Publishing

Impressum/Imprint (nur für Deutschland/ only for Germany)

Bibliografische Information der Deutschen Nationalbibliothek: Die Deutsche Nationalbibliothek verzeichnet diese Publikation in der Deutschen Nationalbibliografie; detaillierte bibliografische Daten sind im Internet über http://dnb.d-nb.de abrufbar.

Alle in diesem Buch genannten Marken und Produktnamen unterliegen warenzeichen-, marken- oder patentrechtlichem Schutz bzw. sind Warenzeichen oder eingetragene Warenzeichen der jeweiligen Inhaber. Die Wiedergabe von Marken, Produktnamen, Gebrauchsnamen, Handelsnamen, Warenbezeichnungen u.s.w. in diesem Werk berechtigt auch ohne besondere Kennzeichnung nicht zu der Annahme, dass solche Namen im Sinne der Warenzeichen- und Markenschutzgesetzgebung als frei zu betrachten wären und daher von jedermann benutzt werden dürften.

Verlag: Lambert Academic Publishing AG & Co. KG
Dudweiler Landstr. 99, 66123 Saarbrücken, Deutschland
Telefon +49 681 3720-310, Telefax +49 681 3720-3109, Email: info@lap-publishing.com

Herstellung in Deutschland:
Schaltungsdienst Lange o.H.G., Berlin
Books on Demand GmbH, Norderstedt
Reha GmbH, Saarbrücken
Amazon Distribution GmbH, Leipzig
ISBN: 978-3-8383-4811-7

Imprint (only for USA, GB)

Bibliographic information published by the Deutsche Nationalbibliothek: The Deutsche Nationalbibliothek lists this publication in the Deutsche Nationalbibliografie; detailed bibliographic data are available in the Internet at http://dnb.d-nb.de.

Any brand names and product names mentioned in this book are subject to trademark, brand or patent protection and are trademarks or registered trademarks of their respective holders. The use of brand names, product names, common names, trade names, product descriptions etc. even without a particular marking in this works is in no way to be construed to mean that such names may be regarded as unrestricted in respect of trademark and brand protection legislation and could thus be used by anyone.

Publisher:
Lambert Academic Publishing AG & Co. KG
Dudweiler Landstr. 99, 66123 Saarbrücken, Germany
Phone +49 681 3720-310, Fax +49 681 3720-3109, Email: info@lap-publishing.com

Printed in the U.S.A.
Printed in the U.K. by (see last page)
ISBN: 978-3-8383-4811-7

CONTENTS

. INTRODUCTION

1. CONTROLLED RELEASE MATRIX SYSTEMS

Controlled release dosage forms are formulated in such a manner so as to make the contained drug available over an extended period of time following administration. Expressions such as controlled-release, prolonged-action, repeat action and sustained-release have also been used to describe such dosage forms. A typical controlled release system is designed to provide constant or nearly constant drug levels in plasma with reduced fluctuations via slow release over an extended period of time. In practical terms, an oral controlled release should allow a reduction in dosing frequency as compared to when the same drug is presented as a conventional dosage form.[31] A matrix device consists of drug dispersed homogenously throughout a polymer matrix. Two major types of materials are used in the preparation of matrix devices.[47]

Hydrophobic carriers:

- Digestible base (fatty compounds) – glycerides - glyceryltristearate, fatty alcohols, fatty acids, waxes - carnauba wax [1]etc.

- Non-digestible base (insoluble plastics) - methylacrylate - ethylmethacrylate, polyvinyl chloride, polyethylene, ethyl cellulose etc.

Hydrophilic polymers:

- Methylcellulose, Sodiumcarboxy methylcellulose, Hydroxypropyl methylcellulose, Sodium alginate, Xanthan gum, Polyethylene oxide and Carbopols.

1.1.1. ADVANTAGES OF THE MATRIX SYSTEMS:

- Easy to manufacture.
- Versatile, effective and low cost.
- Can be made to release high molecular weight compounds.
- Since the drug is mixed in the matrix system, accidental leakage of the total drug component is less likely to occur, although occasionally, cracking of the matrix material can cause unwanted release.

1.1.2. DISADVANTAGES OF THE MATRIX SYSTEMS:

- The remaining matrix must be removed after the drug has been released
- The drug release rates vary with the square root of time. Release rate continuously diminishes due to an increase in diffusional resistance and/or a decrease in effective area at the diffusion front.[31] However, a substantial sustained effect can be produced through the use of very slow release rates, which in many applications are indistinguishable from zero-order.[20]

1.2. MECHANISMS OF DRUG RELEASE FROM MATRIX SYSTEMS

The release of drug from controlled devices is via dissolution of the matrix or diffusion of drug through the matrix or a combination of the two mechanisms.

1.2.1. DISSOLUTION CONTROLLED SYSTEMS

A drug with slow dissolution rate will demonstrate sustaining properties, since the release of the drug will be limited by the rate of dissolution. In principle, it would seem possible to prepare extended release products by decreasing the dissolution rate of drugs that are highly water-soluble. This can be done by:

- Preparing an appropriate salt or derivative
- Coating the drug with a slowly dissolving material – encapsulation dissolution control.
- Incorporating the drug into a tablet with a slowly dissolving carrier – matrix dissolution control (a major disadvantage is that the drug release rate continuously decreases with time).[20]

The dissolution process can be considered diffusion-layer-controlled, where the rate of diffusion from the solid surface to the bulk solution through an unstirred liquid film is the rate-determining step. The dissolution process at steady-state is described by the Noyes-Whitney equation:

$$\frac{dC}{dt} = k_D \cdot A \cdot (C_s - C) = \frac{D}{h} \cdot A \cdot (C_s - C)$$

............Eq-1

dc/d$_t$ - dissolution rate

K_D - the dissolution rate constant (equivalent to the diffusion coefficient divided by the thickness of the diffusion layer D/h)

D - Diffusion coefficient

Cs - Saturation solubility of the solid

C - Concentration of solute in the bulk solution

A - Surface area

Equation-1 predicts that the rate of release can be constant only if the following parameters are held constant: surface area, diffusion coefficient, diffusion layer thickness and concentration difference. However, under normal conditions, it is unlikely that these parameters will remain constant, especially surface area, and this is the case for combination diffusion and dissolution systems.[20]

1.2.2. DIFFUSION CONTROLLED SYSTEMS

Diffusion systems are characterized by the release rate of a drug being dependent on its diffusion through an inert membrane barrier, which is usually a water-insoluble polymer. In general, two types or subclasses of diffusional systems are recognized: reservoir devices and matrix devices[4]. It is very common for the diffusion-controlled devices to exhibit a non-zero order release rate due to an increase in diffusional resistance and a decrease in effective diffusion area as the release proceeds.[47]

1.2.2.1. DIFFUSION IN MATRIX DEVICES

In this model, drug in the outside layer exposed to the bathing solution is dissolved first and then diffuses out of the matrix. This process continues with the interface between the bathing solution and the solid drug moving toward the interior. It follows obviously that for this system to be diffusion controlled, the rate of dissolution of drug particles within the matrix must be much faster than the diffusion rate of dissolved drug leaving the matrix.[20]

3

Derivation of the mathematical model to describe this system involves the following assumptions:

a) A pseudo-steady state is maintained during drug release.

b) The diameter of the drug particles is less than the average distance of drug diffusion through the matrix.

c) The diffusion coefficient of drug in the matrix remains constant (no change occurs in the characteristics of the polymer matrix.

d) The bathing solution provides sink conditions at all times.

e) No interaction occurs between the drug and the matrix.

f) The total amount of drug present per unit volume in the matrix is substantially greater than the saturation solubility of the drug per unit volume in the matrix (excess solute is present) [1]

g) Only the diffusion process occurs.[31]

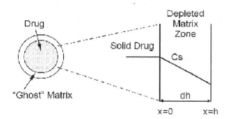

Fig.1 Schematic representation of a matrix release system

For a homogenous monolithic matrix system corresponding to the schematic Figure 1, the release behavior can be described by the following equation:

$$\frac{dM}{dh} = C_0 \cdot dh - \frac{C_s}{2}$$

...............Eq-2

Where,

dM   - Change in the amount of drug released per unit area

dh   - Change in the thickness of the zone of matrix that has been depleted of drug

C_0 - Total amount of drug in a unit volume of matrix

4

$_s$ - Saturated concentration of the drug within the matrix

From diffusion theory:

$$dM = \frac{D_m \cdot C_s}{h} \cdot dt$$

... ...Eq-3

Where,

D_m . is the diffusion coefficient in the matrix

By combining equations (2) and (3):

$$M = [C_s \cdot D_m \cdot (2C_0 - C_s) \cdot t]^{1/2}$$

... ...Eq-4

When the amount of drug is in excess of the saturation concentration, ($C_0 >> C_s$)

$$M = [2C_s \cdot D_m \cdot C_0 \cdot t]^{1/2}$$

... ...Eq-5

That indicates that the amount of drug released is a function of square root of time. Drug release from a porous monolithic matrix involves the simultaneous penetration of surrounding liquid, dissolution of drug and leaching out of the drug through tortuous interstitial channels and pores. The volume and length of the openings must be accounted for in the drug release from a porous or granular matrix:

$$M = [D_s \cdot C_a \cdot \frac{p}{T} \cdot (2C_0 - p \cdot C_a) \cdot t]^{1/2}$$

... ...Eq-6

Where,

   - Porosity of the matrix
   - Tortuosity
$_a$ - Solubility of the drug in the release medium

5

Ds   - Diffusion coefficient in the release medium.

T   -Thickness of the layer

Similarly for pseudo-steady state (C0 >>Cs):

$$M = [2D_s \cdot C_a \cdot C_0 \cdot \frac{p}{T} t]^{1/2}$$

$$\dots\dots\dots\dots..Eq\text{-}7$$

The porosity is the fraction of matrix that exists as pores or channels into which the surrounding liquid can penetrate. It is the total porosity of the matrix after the drug has been extracted; it consists of initial porosity due to the presence of air or void space in the matrix before the leaching process begins as well as the porosity created by extracting the drug and the water-soluble excipients.

$$p = p_a + \frac{C_0}{\rho} + \frac{C_{ex}}{\rho_{ex}}$$

$$\dots\dots\dots\dots.Eq\text{-}8$$

Where ρ is the drug density and ρ_{ex} and C_{ex} are the density and the concentration of water-soluble excipient respectively. In a case where no water-soluble excipient is used in the formulation and initial porosity is much smaller than porosity created by drug extraction, total porosity becomes:

$$p = \frac{C_0}{\rho}$$

$$\dots\dots\dots\dots.Eq\text{-}9$$

Hence the release equations can be written as:

$$M = [D_s \cdot C_a \cdot \frac{p}{T} \cdot (2C_0 - p \cdot C_a) \cdot t]^{1/2}$$

$$\dots\dots\dots\dots.Eq\text{-}6$$

$$M = [2D_s \cdot C_a \cdot C_0 \cdot \frac{p}{T} t]^{1/2}$$

$$\dots\dots\dots\dots.Eq\text{-}10$$

6

or purpose of data treatment, equation (6) can be reduced to

$$M = k \cdot t^{1/2}$$

............Eq-11

Where k is a constant, so that the amount of drug released versus the square root of time will be linear, f the release of drug from matrix is diffusion-controlled. If this is the case, one may control the release f drug from a homogeneous matrix system by varying the following parameters such as:

- Initial concentration of drug in the matrix
- Porosity
- Tortuosity
- Polymer system forming the matrix.
- Solubility of the drug.[1 & 20]

In a hydrophilic matrix, there are two competing mechanisms involved in the drug release: Fickian diffusion release and relaxation release. Diffusion is not the only pathway by which a drug is released from the matrix; the erosion of the matrix following polymer relaxation contributes to the overall release. The relative contribution of each component to the total release is primarily dependent on the properties of a given drug. For example, the release of a sparingly soluble drug from hydrophilic matrices involves the simultaneous absorption of water and desorption of drug via a swelling-controlled diffusion mechanism[31 & 5]. As water penetrates into a glassy polymeric matrix, the polymer swells and its glass transition temperature is lowered. At the same time, the dissolved drug diffuses through this swollen rubbery region into the external releasing medium. This type of diffusion and swelling does not generally follow a Fickian diffusion mechanism. Peppas[39] introduced a semi-empirical equation to describe drug release behaviour from hydrophilic matrix systems:

$$Q = k \cdot t^n$$

$$\dots \dots \dots \text{Eq-12}$$

Where Q is the fraction of drug released in time t, k is the rate constant incorporating characteristics of the macromolecular network system and the drug and n is the diffusional exponent. It has been shown that the value of n is indicative of the drug release mechanism.

For n=0.5, drug release follows a Fickian diffusion mechanism that is driven by a chemical potential gradient.

For n=1 drug release occurs via the relaxation transport that is associated with stresses and phase transition in hydrated polymers.

For 0.5<n<1 non-Fickian diffusion is often observed as a result of the contributions from diffusion and polymer erosion.[31] In order to describe relaxation transport[6], introduced a second term in equation (12):

$$Q = k_1 \cdot t^n + k_2 \cdot t^{2n}$$

$$\dots \dots \dots \text{Eq-13}$$

Where k_1 and k_2 are constants reflecting the relative contributions of Fickian and relaxation mechanisms.

In the case the surface area is fixed, the value of n should be 0.5 and equation (13) becomes:

$$Q = k_1 \cdot t^{0.5} + k_2 \cdot t$$

$$\ldots \ldots \ldots \ldots \text{Eq-14}$$

Where the first and second term represent drug release due to diffusion and polymer erosion, respectively.[31]

1.2.3. BIOERODIBLE AND COMBINATION DIFFUSION AND DISSOLUTION SYSTEMS

Drug release from controlled delivery systems will never be dependent on dissolution or diffusion alone. In practice, the dominant mechanism for release will overshadow other processes enough to allow classification as either dissolution rate-limited or diffusion-controlled release.[20]

Swelling-controlled matrices exhibit a combination of both diffusion and dissolution mechanisms. Here the drug is dispersed in the polymer, but instead of an insoluble or non-erodible polymer, swelling of the polymer occurs. This allows for the entrance of water, which causes dissolution of the drug and diffusion out of the swollen matrix. In these systems the release rate is highly dependent on the polymer-swelling rate and drug solubility. This system usually minimizes burst effects, as rapid polymer swelling occurs before drug release.[20]

With regards to swellable matrix systems, different models have been proposed to describe the diffusion, swelling and dissolution processes involved in the drug release mechanism.[37, 38, 39] however the key element of the drug release mechanism is the forming of a gel layer around the matrix, capable of preventing matrix disintegration and further rapid water penetration.

When a matrix that contains a swellable glassy polymer comes in contact with a solvent or swelling agent, there is an abrupt change from the glassy to the rubbery state, which is associated with the swelling process. The individual polymer chains, originally in the unperturbed state absorb water so that their end to end distance and radius of gyration expand to a new solvated state. This is due to the lowering of the transition temperature of the polymer (Tg), which is controlled by the characteristic concentration of the swelling agent and depends on both temperature and thermodynamic interactions of the polymer– water system.[6] A sharp distinction between the glassy and rubbery regions is observed and the matrix increases in volume because of swelling. On a molecular basis, this phenomenon can activate a convective drug transport, thus increasing the reproducibility of the drug release. The result is an anomalous non-fickian transport of the drug, owing to the polymer-chain relaxation behind the swelling position. This, in turn, creates osmotic stresses and convective transport effects.

The gel strength is important in the matrix performance and is controlled by the concentration, viscosity and chemical structure of the rubbery polymer. This restricts the suitability of the hydrophilic polymers for preparation of swellable matrices. Polymers such as carboxymethyl cellulose, hydroxypropyl cellulose or tragacanth gum, do not form the gel layer quickly. Consequently, they are not recommended as excipients to be used alone in swellable matrices.[15]

The swelling behaviour of heterogeneous swellable matrices is described by front positions, where 'front' indicates the position in the matrix in which the physical conditions sharply change. Three fronts are present, as shown in Figure 2:

- The 'swelling front' clearly separates the rubbery region (with enough water to lower the Tg below the experimental temperature) from the glassy region (where the polymer exhibits a Tg that is above the experimental temperature).

- The 'erosion front', separates the matrix from the solvent. The gel-layer thickness as a function of time is determined by the relative position of the swelling and erosion moving fronts.

- The 'diffusion front' located between the swelling and erosion fronts, and constituting the boundary that separates solid from dissolved drug, has been identified.

- During drug release, the diffusion front position in the gel phase is dependent on drug solubility and loading. The diffusion front movement is also related to drug dissolution rate in the gel.

Fig.2The fronts in a swellable HPMC matrix

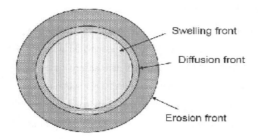

Drug release is controlled by the interaction between water, polymer and drug. The delivery kinetics depends on the drug gradient in the gel layer. Therefore, drug concentration and thickness of the gel layer governs the drug flux.[3] Drug concentration in the gel depends on drug loading and solubility. Gelayer thickness depends on the relative contributions of solvent penetration, chain disentanglement and mass (polymer and drug) transfer in the solvent. Initially solvent penetration is more rapid than chain disentanglement, and a rapid build- up of gel-layer thickness occurs. However, when the solvent penetrates slowly, owing to an increase in the diffusional distance, little change in gel thickness is observed since penetration and disentanglement rates are similar. Thus gel-layer thickness dynamics in wellable matrix tablets exhibit three distinct patterns.

The thickness increases when solvent penetration is the fastest mechanism, and it remains constant when the disentanglement and water penetration occur at a similar rate. Finally, the gel-layer thickness decreases when the entire polymer has undergone the glassy–rubbery transition. In conclusion, the central element of the release mechanism is a gel-layer forming around the matrix in response to water penetration. Phenomena that govern gel-layer formation, and consequently drug-release rate, are water penetration, polymer swelling, drug dissolution and diffusion, and matrix erosion. Drug release is controlled by drug diffusion through the gel layer, which can dissolve and/or erode.

1.3. IMPACT OF FORMULATION & PROCESS VARIABLES ON THE DRUG RELEASE FROM EXTENDED RELEASE MATRIX SYSTEMS.

1.3.1. FORMULATION VARIABLES:

The physicochemical characteristics of the drug, in particular its aqueous solubility, should be considered in the formulation of a matrix system. The following recommendations apply to matrix systems (Table 1):

Table1. Application of matrix for drug delivery systems

Matrix system	Drug delivery mechanism	Drugs not recommended
Hydrophilic		
Swellable / erodible	Diffusion and erosion	Very soluble
Erodible	Erosion	Freely soluble
Hydrophobic		
Monolithic	Diffusion	Practically insoluble
Multiparticulate	Diffusion	Freely soluble
Erodible/Degradable	Erosion/Enzymatic degradation	

Other drug properties affecting system design include drug stability in the system and at the site of absorption, pH-dependent solubility, particle size and specific surface area.

Effect of particle size of drug

Effect of drug particle size on release is important in the case of moderately soluble drugs. Velasco et al.[46] (1999) showed that for a given effective surface area, diclofenac particle size influenced the release rate from hydroxypropyl methyl cellulose (HPMC) tablets. The smallest particle size of drug dissolved more easily when dissolution medium penetrated through the matrix resulting in a greater role for diffusion. The larger particle size dissolved less readily and therefore was more prone to erosion at the matrix surface. A similar dependence was shown for a less soluble drug, indomethacin.[16]

Hogan et al.[19](1989) showed that in the case of water-soluble aminophylline or propranolol HPMC-based tablets an increase in drug particle size did not significantly alter the release rate of the drug. A noticeable effect was seen only at a low drug: HPMC ratio and at a large drug particle size (above 250µm) was seen; in this case, rapid dissolution of the water soluble drug would leave a matrix with low tortuosity and high porosity.

Effect of drug: polymer ratio

For diclofenac tablets formulated with HPMC, Velasco et al.[45](1999) showed that an increase in drug: polymer ratio reduced the release rate. This was because an increase in polymer concentration caused an increase in the viscosity of the gel (by making it more resistant to drug diffusion and erosion) as well as the formation of a gel layer with a longer diffusional path. Similar findings were reported by Lekhi et al.[32](1999) Diffusional release of watersoluble drug metoprolol (primarily controlled by the gel thickness) decreased with increasing HPMC incorporation.

By varying the polymer level (Methocel® K4M 10-40%), Nellore et al.[23](1999) achieved different metoprolol in vitro release profiles.

Sung et al.[41](1996) demonstrated that changes in HPMC: lactose ratio can be used to produce a wide range of drug (adinazolam mesylate) release rates.For Ethocel® 100 and Eudragit® RSPO matrices, Roza et al.(1999) showed that an increase in the polymer content resulted in a decrease in the drug release rates due to a decrease in the total porosity of the matrices (initial porosity plus porosity due to the dissolution of the drug).

Effect of polymer nature

Various grades of commercially available HPMC differ in the relative proportion of the hydroxypropyl and methoxyl substitutions; increasing the amount of hydrophilic hydroxypropyl groups lead to a faster hydration: Methocel®K > Methocel®E > Methocel®F. Generally rapid hydrating Methocel®K grade is preferred, especially for highly soluble drugs where a rapid rate of hydration is necessary. It is important to note that an inadequate polymer hydration rate may lead to dose dumping, due to quick penetration of gastric fluids into the tablet core.[7]

Sung et al.[41](1996) compared different viscosity grades of HPMC (Methocel® K100LV, K15, K100). The fastest release of adinazolam mesilate was achieved for the K100LV formulation. The K4M formulation exhibited a slightly greater drug release than K15M and K100M. Due to the lack of a significant difference in the release profiles between K15M and K100M, the authors suggested a limiting HPMC viscosity of 15000cP, above which if viscosity increased, the release rate would no longer decrease. Similarly, formulations containing higher HPMC viscosity grades had slower HPMC release, but no limiting HPMC viscosity was observed for polymer release.

In each grade, for a fixed polymer level, the viscosity of the selected polymer affects the diffusional and mechanical characteristics of the matrix. By comparing different Methocel®K viscosity grades,

13

Nellore et al.[23](1998) found that the higher viscosity gel layers provided a more tortuous and resistant barrier to diffusion, which resulted in slower release of the drug.

Effect of polymer particle size

Velasco et al.[45](1999) found that the diclofenac sodium release rate from HPMC tablets decreased as the polymer particle increased. Also, as the HPMC particle size increased, the lag period decreased – the drug release occurred during the initial dissolution stage, prior to the formation of the gel layer (coarse fraction of HPMC hydrated slower).

Campos-Aldrete and Villafuerte-Robles (1999) found that increasing particle size of HPMC allowed the free dissolution of metronidazole at higher proportion before the gel was established. Decreasing particle size caused a smaller burst effect and induced lag times. The explanation was based on a faster swelling of the smaller particles that allowed a rapid establishment of the gel barrier.

Heng et al.(2001) observed significant effect of HPMC particle size on aspirin release for polymer concentrations up to 20%. A mean HPMC (Methocel® K15M Premium) particle size of 113μm was identified as a critical threshold for the release of aspirin. The drug release rate increased markedly when polymer particle size was increased above 113μm. The release rate was much less sensitive to changes in particle size below 113μm. The aspirin release mechanism followed first order kinetics, when mean HPMC particle size was below 113μm. The release mechanism deviated from first order kinetics, when the mean particle size was above 113μm. Polymer fractions with similar mean particle size but differing size distributions were also found to influence drug release rates but not the release mechanism.

Effect of fillers

Nellore et al.[23] studied the effect of filler (57% of the tablet weight) on a metoprolol formulation at 20% Methocel® K4M level. They concluded that filler solubility had a limited effect on release rate. The release profiles showed a decrease of about 5-7% after 6h, as the filler was changed from lactose to lactose – microcrystalline cellulose then to dicalcium phosphate dihydrate - microcrystalline cellulose. Addition of soluble fillers enhanced the dissolution of soluble drugs by decreasing the tortuosity of the diffusion path of the drug, while insoluble fillers like dicalcium phosphate dihydrate got entrapped in the matrix. Also, they assumed that presence of a swelling insoluble filler like microcrystalline cellulose changed the release profile to a small extent due to a change in swelling at the tablet surface.

Changing the filler from 100% dicalcium phosphate dihydrate to 100% lactose resulted in an increase in metoprolol release from Methocel® K100LV tablets at 4, 6 and 12h (Rekhi et al).[33] This was explained by dissolution of lactose and the consequent reduction in the tortuosity and or gel strength of the polymer.

Similar dissolution profiles were obtained for filler concentration up to 48%. No dose dumping due to stress cracks.[7] During gelling were observed in the case of insoluble fillers.

Effect of surfactants

Feely and Davis[15] (1988) characterized the ability of charged ionic surfactants to retard the release of oppositely charged drugs from HPMC tablets (chlorphemiramine maleate and sodium alkylsulphates, sodium salicylate and cetylpiridinium bromide). The mechanism involved was an *in situ* drug-surfactant ionic interaction, resulting in a complex with low aqueous solubility, that the release would be more dependent on the matrix erosion than diffusion. The retarding effect was dependent upon the surfactant concentration in the matrix and independent on the surfactant hydrocarbon chain length. The pH of the environment played an important role, by altering the ionization of both the drug and the surfactant. The ionic strength of the dissolution medium affected the action of the resin.

Effect of polymeric excipients

Feely and Davis[15] (1988) studied the effect of polymeric additives (non-ionic polyethylene glycol 6000 or ethyl cellulose, cationic diethylaminoethyl dextran, anionic sodium carboxymethyl cellulose Na-CMC) on drug release (chlorpheniramine maleate, sodium salicylate and potassium phenoxymethylpenicillin) from HPMC matrix (85%). Non-ionic polymers (15% of tablet weight) did not significantly alter the release rates.

Effect of addition of organic acids

In order to overcome the pH dependent release of a weakly basic drug (verapamil HCl) from matrix tablets, Streubel et al. (1986) added organic acids, which were expected to create a constant acidic microenvironment inside the tablets. Substances selected (fumaric, sorbic and adipic acid) had high acidic strength (low pKa value) and relatively low solubility in 0.1N HCl. These acids dissolved rather slowly and remained in the tablets during the entire period of drug release. Independent of the pH of the dissolution medium, the pH inside the tablet was acidic and thus the solubility of the weakly basic drug was high. In addition, at high pH, the organic acids acted as pore formers.

The release rates obtained for both ethyl cellulose and HPMC matrices were pH-independent. Among the three acids, fumaric acid showed the best results, due to the lowest pKa value.

1.3.2. PROCESS VARIABLES

Effect of compression force

It has been reported (Velasco et al. 1999)[46] for HPMC tablets, that although the compression force had a significant effect on tablet hardness, its effect on drug release from HPMC tablets was minimal. It could be assumed that the variation in compression force should be closely related to a change in the porosity of the tablets. However, as the porosity of the hydrated matrix is independent of the initial porosity, the compression force seems to have little influence on drug release. The influence of compression force could only be observed in the lag time (Velasco et al). Tablets made at the lowest crushing strength (compression force 3kN) with Methocel®K4M showed an initial burst effect due to an initial partial disintegration. Once the polymer was swollen, the dissolution profiles became similar to those tablets compressed to a higher crushing strength.

Rekhi et al.[33](1999) reported similar findings, i.e. changes in compression force or crushing strength appeared to have minimal effect on drug release from HPMC matrix tablets once a critical hardness was achieved. Increased dissolution was only observed when the tablets were too soft and it was attributed to the lack of powder compaction or consolidation (3kP).

Effect of tablet shape

Rekhi et al.[33](1999) showed that the size and shape of the tablet for the matrix system undergoing diffusion and erosion might impact the drug dissolution rate.

Modification of the surface area for metoprolol tartarate tablets formulated with Methocel® K100LV from the standard concave shape (0.568sq. in.) to caplet shape (0.747 sq. in.) showed an approximately 20-30% increase in dissolution at each time point. Furthermore, they recommended that for maximum maintenance of controlled release characteristics, tablet matrices should be as near spherical as possible to produce minimum release rate. The release rate of the drug (theophylline) from erodible hydrogel matrix tablets (HPMC E50) having different geometrical shapes (compressed under the same compression force) was found (Karasulu et al] to be the highest on trianglar tablets and successively in order of decreasing amounts on half spherical and cylindrical tablets. This was attributed to heterogenous erosion of the matrices.

16

Effect of tablet size

For tablets having the same aspect ratio and drug concentration, Siepman et al[39] found that the tablet size had a very strong influence on the release rate; within 24 hours, 99.8% was released from the small tablets, 83.1% from the medium size and 50.9% from the large tablets. The explanation was based on the higher surface area referred to the volume for the small tablets than for the large ones. In addition, the diffusion pathways were much longer in large tablets than in small ones. Thus the relative amount of drug released versus time was much higher for small tablets. The variation of the size of the tablet was an effective tool to achieve a desired release.

. OBJECTIVE AND PLAN OF WORK

.1. OBJECTIVE

To develop a Levodopa and Carbidopa controlled release tablets comparable to the marketed formulation.

SPECIFIC AIMS:

1. Preformulation studies involving drug excipients interaction
2. Marketed product evaluation.
3. Development of various formulations with different polymers.
4. Dissolution profile of developed formulations in pH 4.0 acetate buffer.
5. Selection and optimization of the best formulation.
6. Comparison of best formulae with marketed product.
7. Determination of $f2$ (Similarity) factor.
8. To perform stability studies for best formulations.

The rationale for selecting the combination of Levodopa and Carbidopa:

Levodopa and Carbidopa is a medication used to treat Parkinson's disease. Parkinson's disease is believed to be related to low levels of a chemical called dopamine in the brain.
Levodopa is turned into dopamine in the body.
If levodopa alone is administered most of it undergoes peripheral decarboxylation by DOPA decarboxylase, as a result it looses its lipophilicity and can't cross the Blood Brain Barrier. If it is

17

administered in combination with Carbidopa, Carbidopa prevents the peripheral decarboxylation of levodopa so it retains its lipophilicity due to the presence of carboxylic group as such.

2. PLAN OF WORK:

o achieve the desired controlled release tablet formulation of Levodopa and Carbidopa, the xperimental study was framed as follows:

1. Formulation development of diffusion based controlled release matrix tablets of Levodopa and Carbidopa (200 mg +50 mg) using various concentrations of polymers such as HPMCK4M, HPMCK15M and Carbopol 974 P and selection of the optimized formulation.

2. Evaluation of physical parameters such as

   - Weight variation
   - Tablet thickness
   - Tablet hardness
   - Friability
   - Drug content of the matrix tablets
   - Study of *in vitro* drug release profiles in pH 4.0 acetate buffer using USP II Paddle apparatus.
   - Calculation of f_2 factor for the determination of similarity between the developed formulation and marketed formulation.
   - Stability Studies as per ICH guidelines.

3. Comparison studies of drug release from different polymers

3. Material and methods

3.1 Materials: suppliers

The following raw materials and chemicals are used in this work:

S No	Material	Manufacturer & Place
1	Levodopa	Venkar Labs, Hyderabad.
2	Carbidopa	Venkar Labs, Hyderabad.
3	HPMC K4M	Dow chemical company
4	HPMC K15M	Dow chemical company
5	Carbopol 974P	IPS Chemical Company
6	Avicel PH 102	Zydus Cadila
7	Magnesium stearate	S.D. Fine Chemicals Ltd
8	Aerosil	S.D.Fine Chemicals Ltd
9	Talc	S.D. Fine Chemicals Ltd
10	Concentrated hydrochloric acid	Merck limited
11	Potassium dihydrogen phosphate	S.D. chemicals
12	Sodium hydroxide	S.D. Fine Chemicals Ltd
13	Methanol (AR)	Ranbaxy fine chemicals

3.2. EQUIPMENTS:

The instruments and equipments used in the present work were given in following Table

Table2: List of Equipments

S No	Equipment	Make & Model
1	pH Analyzer	Elico
2	Digital Weighing Balance 300grams	AND
3	Digital Weighing scale 6 kg	Essae
4	Mechanical Stirrer I	Remi
5	Mechanical Stirrer II	Remi
6	Refrigerator	Godrej
7	Magnetic Stirrer	Remi
8	Heating mantle	BTI
9	Hot air oven	Yorco
10	Bulk Density Apparatus	Electrolab
11	SS 316 Mesh # 12, 16, 20, 40, 60 & 100	Prathibha
12	Digital Tablet Dissolution Test Apparatus	LABINDIA-DISSO-2000
13	UV/VIS spectrophotometer	Perkin-Elmer- lambda 25
14	HPLC (UVD340U)	Dionex
15	HPLC	Perkin Elmer,
16	Tablet Hardness tester	Dr Schleunger
17	Friability Tester	Electrolab
18	Compression Machine	Chamunda
19	Tray Dryer	Chamunda
20	Stability Chamber $25^{O}C$ / 60% RH	Thermolab
21	Stability Chamber $40^{O}C$ / 75% RH	Thermolab
22	Photostability Chamber	Thermolab

3.3.   DRUG PROFILES:

3.3.1. LEVODOPA:

Description   : Levodopa is a white or creamy white crystalline powder,   which is odorless and bitter taste.

Chemical Name   : L-α-amino-β-(3, 4, dihydrobenzene)-propionic acid.

Structure   :

Molecular Formula   : $C_9H_{11}NO_4$
Molecular Weight   : 197.2
Solubility   : Slightly soluble in water & readily soluble in dil HCl.
Melting Point   : 276 to 278°C.
pH of 1% solution   : 5.5 to 6.0
Spectrophotometry : UV detection at 280 nm

CLINICAL PHARMACOLOGY:

Mechanism of Action   : Levodopa is a metabolic precursor of dopamine and it acts by augmenting the effectiveness of remaining nigrostriatal neurons.

Uses	: Used in the treatment of Rigidity, Tremor, Bradykinesia, Gait, Hypomimia and Micrographia.
Absorption	: Absorbed throughout GIT
Half Life	: 2 hours.
Cmax	: 1.7±0.8 µg/ml
Tmax	: 1.4±0.7 hr
Metabolism	:Decarboxylation by DOPA decarboxylase and O- methylation by (Catechol O-Methylase Transferase) COMT.
Storage	: Store in a cool and dry place at 25°C
Stability	: Levodopa is a little heat sensitive drug
Dosage	: Start with 250 mg daily after a meal increasing slowly by 250 mg increments over 3-4 days till maximum therapeutic response is achieved. Maximum 1-8 g daily in divided doses.

3.3.2. CARBIDOPA:

Description   : Carbidopa is a creamy white crystalline powder, odorless and has bitter taste.

Chemical Name   : Benzene propionic acid, α-hydrazino-3,4,-dihydroxy- α-methyl-monohydrate.

Structure:

Molecular Formula   : $C_{10}N_{14}O_4$

Molecular Weight   : 244.3

Solubility   : Slightly soluble in water but readily soluble in dil HCl.

Melting Point   : 206 to 208°C.

Spectrophotometry   : U.V. detection at 282nm

CLINICAL PHARMACOLOGY:

Mechanism of Action   : Peripheral DOPA decarboxylase inhibitor.

Uses   : Used to treat Parkinsonism with Levodoa

Absorption   : Absorbed throughout GIT

Half life   : 2 hours.

Peak Conc   : 1.7±0.8 μg/ml

Peak time   : 1.4±0.7 hr

Metabolism   : By deamination and methylation

Storage   : Store in a cool and dry place at 25°C

4. POLYMER PROFILES:

4.1. HYDROXY PROPYL METHYL CELLULOSE

ydroxy propyl methylcellulose is mixed alkyl cellulose ether and may be regarded as the propylene ycol ether of methyl cellulose.

hemical name : Cellulose, 2-hydroxy propyl methyl ether.

ommon names : Hyperomellose, Methocel

escription : It is an odorless creamy – white, fibrous or granular powder.

olubility : Soluble in cold water, forming a viscous colloidal solution, insoluble in alcohol, ether and chloroform.

H : 6.0 - 8.0 (1% aqueous solution)

el point : 50 to 90°C

ensity : 0.25 to 0.70 g/cm^3

iscosity (mPa s) : 80-120(K100LV), 3000-5600(K4M), 11250-21000(K15M), 80000-120000(K100M).

ability : Very stable in dry conditions. Solutions are stable at pH 3.0-11.0. Aqueous solutions are liable to be effected by microbes.

ses : Suspending agent, Viscosity modifier, Film and matrix forming material, Tablet binder and adhesive ointment ingredient.

3.4.2. CARBOPOL 974P

Carbomers are synthetic high molecular weight polymers of acrylic acids that are cross linked with either allyl sucrose or allyl ether of pentaerythritol.

Common names : Acritamer, acrylic acid polymer, Carbopol, Carboxy

polymethylene, Polyacrylic acid, Pemulen, Ultrez.

Description : It is a white colored fluffy, acidic, hygroscopic powder with slight characteristic odor.

Solubility : Soluble in water, ethanol (95%) and glycerine.

pH : 2.5 - 3.0 (1% aqueous solution)

Gel point : 100 to 105°C

Density : 1.4 g/cm^3

Viscosity : 4000 to 39,400 mPa s.

Stability : Stable, hygroscopic materials that may be heated at temp below 104^{0}C for up to 2 hrs without affecting their thickening efficiency.

Uses : Bioadhesive, Emulsifying agent, Release modifying agent, Suspending agent, Viscosity modifier and Tablet binder.

3.5. PREFORMULATION STUDIES:

3.5.1. Drug-Excipient compatibility:

Drug excipient testing is an investigation of physical and chemical properties of a drug substance alone and when combined with excipients. It is the first step in the rational development of dosage form. The use of Preformulation parameters maximizes the chances in formulating an acceptable, safe, efficacious and stable product.

In this study active pharmaceutical ingredient and different types of excipients are mixed and stored at three different conditions, namely 40°C ± 2°C /75 ± 5%RH; 25°C ± 2°C /60 ± 5%RH; and Photo stability. Physical observations of the blend are recorded during the study at regular interval of one week. Further the samples are required to be assayed.

3.5.2 Evaluation of Levodopa and Carbidopa Granules Properties:

During granulation, after drying and the final the granules or blend were subjected to the following tests.

Loss on drying:

Determination of loss on drying of granules is important. Drying time during granulation is optimized on the LOD value. LOD of each batches are tested at 60°C temperature by using Sartorious electronic LOD apparatus.

Determination of bulk density and tapped density:

An accurately weighed quantity of the powder (W) is carefully poured into the graduated cylinder and volume (V_o) is measured. Then the graduated cylinder was closed with lid, set into the density determination apparatus (bulk density apparatus). The density apparatus is set for 100 taps and after that the volume (V_f) is measured and continued operation till the two consecutive reading are equal. The bulk density and tapped density are calculated using the following formulae.

Bulk density $= W/ V_o$

Tapped density $= W/ V_f$

Where, W= weight of the powder, V_o= initial volume, V_f= final volume

Hausner Ratio:

It indicates the flow properties of the powder and measured by the ratio of tapped density to bulk density.

Hausner Ratio = Tapped Density/ Bulk Density

27

Table 3: **Flow Properties (Hausner ratio)**

S No	Hausner Ratio	Properties
1	0-1.2	Free Flowing
2	1.2-1.6	Cohesive powder

Compressibility index:

It is an important measure of powders, and is obtained from the bulk and tapped densities using the following formula.

The relationship of Carr's indices to flow behaviour of powders is shown in the following table.

$$CI = 100 \ (V_o - V_f) / V_o$$

Table 4: **Flow Properties (Carr's Indices)**

S No	Carr's Indices	Flow Properties
1	5-12	Free-Flowing
2	12-16	Good
3	18-21	Fair
4	23-35	Poor
5	33-38	Very poor
6	>40	Extremely poor

3.5.3. Standard graphs of Levodopa and Carbidopa

Standard graph of Levodopa:

An accurately weighed amount of 100 mg of Levodopa was transferred into a 100 ml volumetric flask. 10 ml of 0.1 H_3PO_4 was added to dissolve the drug and volume made up to 100 ml with deionized water, serial dilutions were made to give concentration of Levodopa ranging from 50µg/ml - 250µg/ml.

he volumetric solutions were scanned in a HPLC to determine the λ max (280 nm) of the drug. The PLC conditions were maintained as described in the section 3.7.1.   The peak areas of the olumetric solutions were recorded at λ max of the drug after a retention time of 3.5 minutes and lotted graphically to give the standard graph of Levodopa.

tandard graph of Carbidopa:

.n accurately weighed amount of 25 mg of Carbidopa was transferred into a 100 ml volumetric flask. 0 ml of 0.1 H_3PO_4 was added to dissolve the drug and volume made up to 100 ml with deionized ater, necessary dilutions were made to give concentration of Carbidopa ranging from 10µg/ml - 0µg/ml.

he volumetric solutions were scanned in a HPLC to determine the λ max (280 nm) of the drug. The eak areas of the volumetric solutions were recorded at λ max of the drug after a retention time of 11.5 inutes and plotted graphically to give the standard graph of Carbidopa.

.5.4. Assay of API

ssay of Levodopa:

evodopa standard solution:

Jeigh accurately 0.0998 g of Levodopa WRS into a 100 ml volumetric flask, and add 10 ml of 0.1M 3P04. Heat and sonicate to dissolve the contents completely. Make up the volume with water up to 00 and mix.

ample preparation:

Jeigh and finely powder 20 tablets to uniform fine powder and transfer an accurately weighed uantity of the powder of about 0.160 g into a 100 ml volumetric flask and add 10 ml of 0.1M H3P04. eat and sonicate to dissolve the contents completely. Makeup the volume with water up to 100 ml and ix it well.

ssay of Carbidopa:

Carbidopa standard solution:

Weigh accurately 0.0256 g of Carbidopa WRS into a 100 ml volumetric flask, and add 10 ml of 0.1M H_3PO_4. Heat and sonicate to dissolve the contents completely. Makeup the volume with water up to 100 and mix.

6. FORMULATION METHODS:

6.1. Procedure for the preparation of tablets by direct compression.

All the ingredients are weighed and sifted through # 40 mesh

All the ingredients are mixed geometrically in a poly bag.

All these ingredients are mixed well for 5-10 min.

The above blend is compressed into tablets with 12mm flat circular shaped punches.

6.2 Procedure for the preparation of tablets by aqueous granulation method.

All the ingredients are accurately weighed and sifted through # 40 mesh except Brilliant blue which is passed through #100 mesh.

Levodopa, Carbidopa, HPMCK4M, Starch and Brilliant blue are mixed well for 5-10 min geometrically in a poly bag.

The above mix is granulated with Povidone K30 dissolved in water or water alone using as granulating fluid. The granules are kept for drying in hot air oven.

Lubricants are mixed with dried granules and mixed well for 5 min.

This blend is compressed using 12 mm flat, round shaped punches.

7. Evaluation of Levodopa and Carbidopa CR Tablets:

uring Compression and after the completion of the compression, the tablets are selected randomly and bjected to the following tests.

ablet weight variation: Select randomly twenty tablets and are individually weighed and the average eight and standard deviation is reported. The weight variation tolerances for uncoated tablets as per SP and IP were given in the Table 5.

able 5: Weight variation tolerances for uncoated tablets

Maximum % difference allowed	Average Weight of tablets (mg)	
	USP XXVII	IP 1996
10	130 or less	80 or less
7.5	130-324	80-250
5	More than 324	More than 250

Hardness: Hardness is determined for 10 tablets of known weight and thickness. The average hardness and standard deviation is reported.

Thickness: Thickness is determined for 20 pre-weighed tablets of each batch using a digital vernier scale and the average thickness and standard deviation are reported.

Friability:

Tablet hardness is not an absolute indicator of strength since some formulations, when compressed into very hard tablets, tend to "cap" or break/chip on attrition. In friability testing, the tablets are subjected to abrasion and shock. A pre weighed tablet sample is placed in the friabilator, which is then operated for 100 revolutions. The tablets are then dedusted and reweighed. The friability limit is NMT 1%.

Friability = Wo-Wf/Wo X 100

Where,

Wo= Initial Weight of tablets

Wf= Final weight of tablets

3.7.1. Dissolution studies (*In vitro* drug release):

Six prepared tablets of Levodopa and Carbidopa (200mg+50mg) are used for the study. The USFDA in its guidance to industry for developing an *in vitro in vivo* correlation for a Controlled Release product, specified the use of pH 4.0 acetate buffer as a dissolution medium.

In vitro drug release was performed for the manufactured tablets according to the USP "Dissolution procedure," over a 12-hour period, using an automated sampling dissolution system. A minimum of 6 tablets per batch were tested.

In vitro drug release is performed for the manufactured tablets over a 12- hour period, using digital tablet dissolution test apparatus LABINDIA-DISSO-2000. Drug release from each tablet was determined by HPLC at 280 nm.

Dissolution method by HPLC:

Identification of samples: Sample peaks are identified based on the known retention times.

Sample preparation:

Apparatus	:	USP Type-II (Paddle)
Medium	:	pH 4.0 Acetate buffer
Volume	:	900 ml
Speed	:	50 RPM
Time	:	1, 2, 4, 6, 12 hours
Temperature	:	37 ±0.5°C

Levodopa standard preparation:

An accurately weighed sample of 0.2199g of Levodopa WRS is taken into a 100 ml volumetric flask, and added 10 ml of O.1M H_3PO_4 and heated and sonicated to dissolve the contents completely. Made up the volume with water up to 100 and mixed well. About 5 ml of this solution is diluted to 50 ml with dissolution medium.

Sample preparation:

One tablet is placed in each dissolution basket containing 900ml of pH 4.0 Acetate buffer in each bowl. Apparatus is run for 12 hours and 5 ml samples are collected at 1, 2, 4, 6, and 12 hr intervals. The sample volume is replaced.

Chromatographic conditions:

Apparatus	:	HPLC
Column	:	C8, 150x4.6mm, 5 micron
Wave length	:	280 nm
Flow rate	:	1 ml/minute
Temperature	:	Ambient
Injection volume	:	20μl

Mobile phase: it is prepared by dissolving 16.5 g of dihydrogen phosphate in 980 ml of water. To this 0.1ml of EDTA, 20 ml of methanol and 1.2 ml of 0.5 M sodium hexane sulfonate are added and finally adjusted the p^H to 3.4 with 1M Ortho phosphoric acid.

Both standard and test samples are filtered and 20 μl of each is injected into HPLC. Peaks are recorded and areas are calculated for both Levodopa and Carbidopa.

The release of Levodopa and Carbidopa in percentage with respect to label claim using following expression.

$$\frac{AT}{AS} \times \frac{WS}{100} \times \frac{5}{250} \times \frac{5}{10} \times \frac{500}{1} \times \frac{10}{5} \times \frac{P}{100} \times \frac{100}{2} \times 1000$$

Where AS & AT are the average peak areas for standard and test preparations correspond to either of Levodopa or Carbidopa, WS is the weight of Levodopa or Carbidopa and P is the percent purity of Levodopa or Carbidopa.

4. Experimental

4.1. Preformulation studies: Certain preformulation studies like drug-excipient compatibility, granules properties were carried out as per the procedures mentioned in the section (3.5).

4.2. Standard graphs for Levodopa and Carbidopa were plotted as per the procedures mentioned in the section (3.5.3).

4.3. Different formulations were prepared using various polymers as per the procedures mentioned in the section (3.6).

4.3.1. Optimization of formula with HPMCK15M by direct compression method

Direct compression technique was used to prepare these formulations as per the procedure mentioned in the section (3.6.1). Polymer HPMCK15M concentration was varied in all the formulae and to compensate the weight difference MCC was used as filler, while the other excipients were maintained constant. The prepared tablets were subjected to different tests namely weight variation, friability, hardness, thickness, assay and *in vitro* dissolution as described previously in the section (3.7).

Table: 6 Comparison of tablets formulated with HPMCK15M

Ingredients	Weight in milligrams per tablet			
	DK15-1	DK15-2	DK15-3	DK15-4
Levodopa	200.00	200.00	200.00	200.00
Carbidopa	50.00	50.00	50.00	50.00
HPMC K 15 M	60.00	50.00	40.00	30.00
MCC	81.10	91.10	101.10	111.10
Ascorbic Acid	0.40	0.40	0.40	0.40
Talc	2.50	2.50	2.50	2.50
Aerosil	2.50	2.50	2.50	2.50
Mg.stearate	3.50	3.50	3.50	3.50
Total	400.00	400.00	400.00	400.00

4.3.2. Optimization of formula with HPMCK4M by aqueous granulation method

Four tablet compositions were used in different trials and four formulae were given in the following table. Direct compression technique was used to prepare these formulations, namely DK4-1 to DK4-5. Final tablet weight was maintained to 400 mg. Polymer HPMCK4M concentration was varied in all the formulae and to compensate the weight difference MCC was used as filler, while the other excipients were maintained constant. The prepared tablets were subjected to different tests namely weight variation, friability, hardness, thickness, assay and *in vitro* dissolution as described previously in the section (3.7).

Table: 7 Comparison of tablets formulated with HPMCK4M

Ingredients	Weight in milligrams per tablet				
	DK4-1	DK4-2	DK4-3	DK4-4	DK4-5
Levodopa	200.00	200.00	200.00	200.00	200.00
Carbidopa	50.00	50.00	50.00	50.00	50.00
HPMC K 4 M	72.00	60.00	48.00	36.00	30.00
MCC	13.00	33.00	53.00	73.00	83.00
Brilliant blue	0.10	0.10	0.10	0.10	0.10
Ascorbic Acid	0.40	0.40	0.40	0.40	0.40
Povidone	8.00	8.00	8.00	8.00	8.00
Water	q.s.	q.s.	q.s.	q.s.	q.s.
HPMC K 4 M	48.00	40.00	32.00	24.00	20.00
Talc	2.50	2.50	2.50	2.50	2.50
Aerosil	2.50	2.50	2.50	2.50	2.50
Mg. stearate	3.50	3.50	3.50	3.50	3.50
Total	400.00	400.00	400.00	400.00	400.00

3.3. Optimization of formula with Carbopol 974P by direct compression method

our tablet compositions were used in different trials and four formulae were given in the following ble. Direct compression technique was used to prepare these formulations, namely DC-1 to DC-4. nal tablet weight was maintained to 400 mg. Polymer Carbopol 974P concentration was varied in all e formulae and to compensate the weight difference MCC was used as filler, while the other cipients were maintained constant. The prepared tablets were subjected to different tests namely eight variation, friability, hardness, thickness, assay and *in vitro* dissolution as described previously the section (3.7).

able: 8   Comparison of tablets formulated with Carbopol 974P

Ingredients	Weight in milligrams per tablet			
	DC-1	DC-2	DC-3	DC-4
Levodopa	200.00	200.00	200.00	200.00
Carbidopa	50.00	50.00	50.00	50.00
Carbopol 974P	70.00	60.00	50.00	40.00
MCC	31.00	41.00	51.00	61.00
Brilliant blue	0.10	0.10	0.10	0.10
Ascorbic Acid	0.40	0.40	0.40	0.40
Talc	2.50	2.50	2.50	2.50
Aerosil	2.50	2.50	2.50	2.50
Mg. stearate	3.50	3.50	3.50	3.50
Total	400.00	400.00	400.00	400.00

4.4. Evaluation of Levodopa and Carbidopa CR Tablets:

The prepared tablets were subjected to different tests namely weight variation, friability, hardness, thickness, assay and *in vitro* dissolution as described previously in the section (3.7).

4.5. Preparation and evaluation of stability batches

Three optimized formulae namely DK15-4, DK4-3, DC-4 were prepared as 3000 tablets per batch as per the procedures mentioned in the respective sections (3.6.1 & 3.6.2). Tablets were evaluated for weight variation, hardness, thickness, friability and drug content as per the procedures mentioned in the section (3.7).

5. RESULTS AND DISCUSSION:

5.1. Preformulation studies

5.1.1. Evaluation of API:

Active Pharmaceutical Ingredient were analysed and the results are tabulated in the following Tables.

Table:9 (a)   **Levodopa API Characterization:**

S No	Test	Results	Specification
1	Description	White to creamy odourless powder	White to creamy odourless powder
2	Solubility	Complies	Slightly soluble in water. Freely soluble in dil HCl
3	Moisture Content	6.5 % w/w	6.9 to 7.9 % w/w
4	Assay by HPLC	99.76%	98 % to 102 %
5	Bulk density	0.5 gm/ml	0.35 to 0.65 gm/ml
6	Tapped density	0.83 gm/ml	0.75 to 0.95 gm/ml

Table:9 (b)   **Carbidopa API Characterization:**

S No	Test	Results	Specification
1	Description	White to creamy odourless powder	White to creamy odourless powder
2	Solubility	Complies	Slightly soluble in water. Freely soluble in 3 N HCl
3	Moisture Content	6.7 % w/w	6.5 to 7.4 % w/w
4	Assay by HPLC	99.76%	98 % to 102 %
5	Bulk density	0.5 gm/ml	0.35 to 0.65 gm/ml
6	Tapped density	0.83 gm/ml	0.75 to 0.95 gm/ml

The results present in the tables 9(a) & 9(b) indicated that the drugs used in the tablet formulations fulfilled all the specifications mentioned in the certificate of analysis of both the drugs.

5.1.3. Determination of physical properties of Levodopa and Carbidopa

Table:10

S.No	Parameter	Levodopa	Carbidopa
1	LOD	0.62	0.85
2	Angle of repose	46^0	48^0
3	Bulk density (g/ml)	0.50	0.31
4	Tapped density (g/ml)	0.83	0.50
5	Compressibility index	21	22
6	Hausner ratio	1.60	1.62

The tabled physical properties are determined for the drug as well as the granules to know the strategy of both the drugs and granules regarding the flow properties as per the procedures mentioned in the section (3.5.2.).

The Compressibility index and Hausner ratio indicated poor flow characteristics. So it was decided to improve the flow properties by inclusion of suitable amounts of lubricants and glidants.

The granules were prepared as per the methods described in the section (3.6.2).

The various parameters like LOD %w/w, Bulk Density, Tapped Density, Compressibility index (%), Angle of Repose and Hausner Ratio were found by the methods as described in the section (3.5.2).

Table: 11   Physical properties of granules :(DK15-4 – DK4-5)

lation	LOD %w/w	Bulk Density	Tapped Density	Compressibility index (%)	Angle of Repose	Hausner Ratio
5-4	0.82	0.398	0.493	19	32^0	1.23
4-1	0.74	0.368	0.479	20	32^0	1.30
4-2	0.83	0.378	0.482	16	30^0	1.27
4-3	0.96	0.382	0.494	15	30^0	1.29
4-4	0.73	0.369	0.496	15	30^0	1.34
4-5	0.90	0.369	0.475	15	30^0	1.28

.2. Standard graphs of Levodopa and Carbidopa

Table:12

Levodopa		Carbidopa	
Conc.(mcg/ml)	Peak area	Conc.(mcg/ml)	Peak area
0	0	0	0
50	756426	10	112576
100	1401831	20	231957
150	2016246	30	325631
200	2701861	40	465912
250	3297096	50	545271
-	-	60	681976

he standard graphs of Levodopa and Carbidopa in deionised water were plotted as shown in figures 3
: 4. The result shows good linearity with a correlation coefficient of 0.9981 and 0.9978 respectively
or Levodopa and Carbidopa.

Fig.3 Standard graph of Levodopa

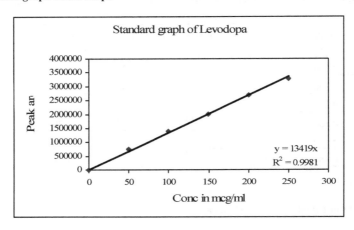

Fig.4 Standard graph of Carbidopa

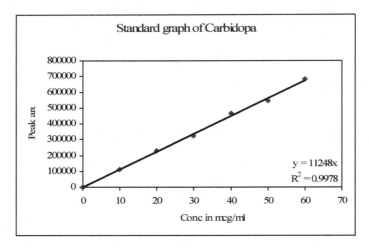

3. Determination of *In vitro* release of drug from marketed formulation SYNDOPA:

Table:13

Time in hrs	% Drug release	
	Levodopa	Carbidopa
0	0	0
1	14.91±0.34	16.49±0.25
2	29.93±0.52	32.78±0.31
4	55.21±0.44	57.28±0.42
6	74.98±0.36	77.53±0.37
12	99.85±0.15	98.36±.018

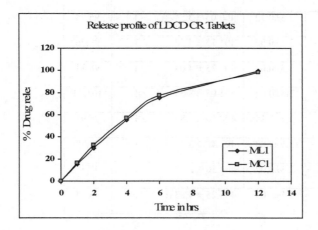

Fig.5 Cumulative drug release profile (Levodopa & Carbidopa) from marketed tablets

The release profiles of both the drugs in the marketed preparation are very close and follow similar path length. The drugs were releasing for 12 hrs and follow approximately zero order release.

Fig.5 Cumulative drug release profile from marketed tablets (syndopa).

4. Evaluation of the prepared formulations:

The prepared tablets from different batches were subjected to weight variation, tablet thickness, tablet hardness, friability and % drug content tests as described in the section 3.7. Tablets of all the batches

43

were within pharmacopoeial limits of 5% weight variation, 5 ± 0.5 Kg/cm^2. Friability and drug content are well within the permissible pharmacopoeial limits.

Table: 14

Formula code	Hardness (Kg/cm^2)	Thickness (mm)	Weight variation (mg)	Friability (%)	Drug content (%)
DK15-1	5± 0.5	3.5±0.06	402.05 ±5.54	<1	95.26
DK15-2	5± 0.5	3.5±0.13	403.40 ± 4.02	<1	98.96
DK15-3	5± 0.5	3.5±0.08	404.45 ± 3.35	<1	96.33
DK15-4	5± 0.5	3.5±0.04	401.00 ± 4.06	<1	97.32
DK4-1	5± 0.5	3.5±0.10	401.50 ± 2.74	<1	98.65
DK4-2	5± 0.5	3.5±0.12	400.05 ± 3.54	<1	96.54
DK4-3	5± 0.5	3.5±0.09	401.75 ± 4.32	<1	99.76
DK4-4	5± 0.5	3.5±0.02	402.75 ± 4.04	<1	98.21
DK4-5	5± 0.5	3.5±0.07	401.05 ± 3.54	<1	101.23
DC-1	5± 0.5	3.5±0.15	400.50 ± 3.84	<1	95.91
DC-2	5± 0.5	3.5±0.08	403.40 ± 3.28	<1	98.79
DC-3	5± 0.5	3.5±0.07	404.50 ± 2.74	<1	97.41
DC-4	5± 0.5	3.5±0.03	403.25 ± 4.23	<1	96.24

5.4.1. *In vitro* Dissolution profiles of Levodopa and Carbidopa CR tablets prepared by direct compression (DK15-1- DK15-4):

Cumulative % drug release from the tablets prepared using polymer HPMC K15M

Table: 15(a)

Time in hrs	Cumulative % drug release of Levodopa			
	DK15-1	DK15-2	DK15-3	DK15-4
0	0	0	0	0
1	4.6±1.21	6.23±2.02	8.57±2.48	19.87±2.23
2	6.83±1.34	11.21±2.47	23.21±3.32	36.25±1.97
4	12.76±2.56	21.32±2.89	31.26±3.64	51.67±2.32
6	19.05±2.42	30.11±3.53	40.08±4.53	63.94±2.17
12	45.24±3.32	57.35±4.31	72.41±4.76	98.38±1.73

Table: 15(b)

Time in hrs	Cumulative % drug release of Carbidopa			
	DK15-1	DK15-2	DK15-3	DK15-4
0	0	0	0	0
1	4.8±1.23	5.45±2.43	7.43±2.86	19.13±1.91
2	6.72±1.67	10.23±3.24	21.12±3.12	34.87±2.27
4	12.65±2.87	19.85±3.68	31.05±4.35	49.92±2.61
6	20.11±3.85	28.24±4.54	39.56±4.87	64.24±1.94
12	44.65±3.74	57.1±5.03	68.56±5.43	97.12±2.25

Fig.6 Cumulative % drug release of Levodopa

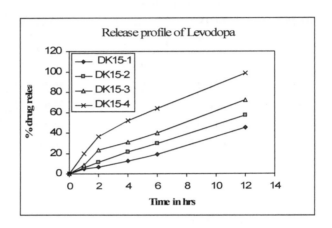

Fig.7 Cumulative % drug release of Carbidopa

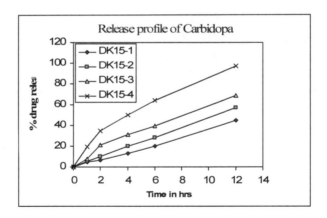

DK15-1 :15%HPMCK15M

DK15-2 :12.5%HPMCK15M

DK15-3 :10%HPMCK15M

DK15-4 :7.5%HPMCK15M

e results of *in vitro* release from HPMC K15M matrix tablets were shown in tables 15(a) & 15(b) d figures 6 & 7. All the formulations except DK15-4 release less than 70% of drug with in12 hrs due higher concentration of polymer. The formulation DK15-4 released more than 95% of the drug in 12 s. However at various time intervals also, the cumulative % drug release is very close to the one from arket. Hence the formulation DK15-4 was selected as optimized formulation. The *f2* values for K15-4 against marketed product were found to be 65 and 69 respectively for Levodopa and arbidopa.

5.4.2. *In vitro* Dissolution profiles of Levodopa and Carbidopa CR tablets prepared by wet granulation (DK4-1- DK4-5):

Cumulative % drug release from the tablets prepared using polymer HPMC K4M

Table 16(a):

Time	Cumulative % drug release of Levodopa				
in hrs	DK4-1	DK4-2	DK4-3	DK4-4	DK4-5
0	0	0	0	0	0
1	5.63±3.56	11.96±3.69	14.34±2.16	17.57±3.08	30.12±3.77
2	14.02±4.37	19.56±4.58	24.86±2.42	32.56±3.57	49.25±4.05
4	24.62±4.74	36.24±4.91	40.12±3.04	60.35±2.98	78.02±3.96
6	36.34±5.07	48.57±5.21	60.89±2.44	82.47±3.67	96.72±4.47
12	61.86±4.83	82.95±3.64	98.97±2.51	99.86±3.80	101.01±4.83

Table: 16(b)

Time	Cumulative % drug release of Carbidopa				
in hrs	DK4-1	DK4-2	DK4-3	DK4-4	DK4-5
0	0	0	0	0	0
1	4.51±3.23	10.75±3.50	13.85±2.52	16.85±2.89	28.92±3.83
2	13.61±4.12	18.87±4.34	23.76±2.07	31.25±3.45	48.68±3.71
4	22.76±3.96	35.56±4.35	39.39±3.16	58.85±2.96	77.64±4.81
6	35.56±5.25	47.34±5.20	59.58±2.51	81.38±4.37	94.89±4.69
12	60.45±4.77	81.66±3.86	97.85±3.05	98.77±3.68	99.97±4.76

.8 Cumulative % drug release of Levodopa

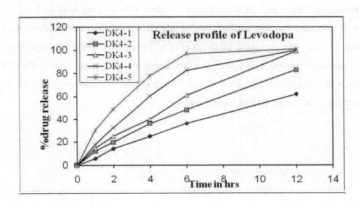

g.9 Cumulative % drug release of Carbidopa

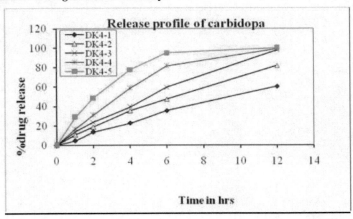

K4-1 : 30%HPMCK4M

K4-2 : 25%HPMCK4M

K4-3 : 20%HPMCK4M

K4-4 : 15%HPMCK4M

K4-5: 12.5%HPMCK4M

The results of *in vitro* release from HPMC K4M matrix tablets are shown in tables 16(a) & 16(b) and figures 8 & 9. Formulations DK4-1 and DK4-2 released less than 85% of drug with in12 hrs due to higher concentration of polymer. The formulations DK4-4 and DK4-5 released more than 95% of the drug within 8 hrs due to lower concentration of polymer. The formulation DK4-3 exhibited similar release profile to the marketed product which was also confirmed by its *f2* factor. Hence this DK4-3 was considered as the best formulation. The *f2* values for DK4-3 against marketed product were found to be 75 and 73 respectively for Levodopa and Carbidopa.

.4.3. *In vitro* Dissolution profiles of Levodopa and Carbidopa CR tablets prepared by direct ompression (DC-1- DC-4):

Table: 17(a)

Time in hrs	Cumulative % drug release of Levodopa			
	DC-1	DC-2	DC-3	DC-4
0	0	0	0	0
1	5.63±2.05	8.26±3.45	18.27±2.12	24.35±2.16
2	10.04±2.58	12.03±3.68	30.65±3.42	34.66±2.07
4	14.64±3.45	24.34±3.74	44.08±3.27	56.68±1.36
6	23.08±3.27	34.43±4.12	54.47±4.03	70.12±2.65
12	34.36±4.04	58.46±4.59	72.58±3.74	100.28±1.72

Table: 17(b)

Time in hrs	Cumulative % drug release of Carbidopa			
	DC-1	DC-2	DC-3	DC-4
0	0	0	0	0
1	4.95±1.96	7.97±3.26	18.31±2.11	23.58±2.14
2	8.12±2.23	12.8±3.51	29.88±3.36	33.67±2.31
4	13.56±3.35	25.12±3.78	43.16±3.69	55.85±1.94
6	22.76±3.52	34.12±4.37	53.74±4.25	70.04±2.43
12	33.25±4.51	57.37±4.82	72.04±3.73	99.88±1.89

Fig.10 Cumulative % drug release of Levodopa

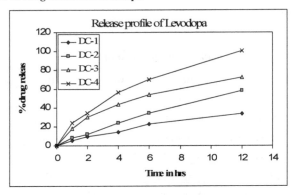

Fig.11 Cumulative % drug release of Carbidopa

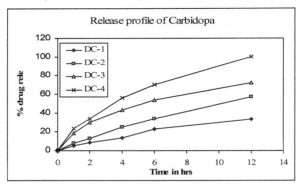

DC-1:17.5%Carbopol974P

DC-2:15%Carbopol974P

DC-3:12.5%Carbopol974P

DC-4:10%Carbopol974P

he results of *in vitro* release from Carbopol 974P matrix tablets are shown in above tables 17(a) & 7(b) and figures 10 & 11. All the formulations except DC-4 released less than 75% of drug within 12 rs due to higher concentration of polymer. The formulation DC-4 released more than 95% of the drug ithin 12 hrs. The formulation DC-4 showed similar release profile to the marketed product which was so confirmed by its similarity factor *f2*. Hence the DC-4 formula was found to be optimized and omparable to the marketed formulation. The *f2* values for DK15-4 against marketed product were und to be 70 and 66 respectively for Levodopa and Carbidopa.

5.5. Comparison of cumulative % drug released from the best formulae

Table: 18

Time	Cumulative % drug released from the best formulae					
	DK15-4		DK4-3		DC-4	
(hrs)	Levodopa	Carbidopa	Levodopa	Carbidopa	Levodopa	Carbidopa
0	0	0	0	0	0	0
1	20.11±2.25	18.65±2.14	14.34±2.16	13.85±2.52	24.35±2.16	23.58±2.14
2	36.56±2.06	35.27±1.87	24.86±2.42	23.76±2.07	34.66±2.07	33.67±2.31
4	52.37±1.98	50.87±2.31	40.12±3.04	39.39±3.16	56.68±1.36	55.85±1.94
6	64.23±2.35	63.54±1.88	60.89±2.44	59.58±2.51	70.12±2.65	70.04±2.43
12	97.78±1.84	96.25±2.34	98.97±2.51	97.85±3.05	100.28±1.72	99.88±1.89

Table: 19

f_1 and f_2 factors of the optimized formulations.

Formulation	Levodopa		Carbidopa	
code	f_1	f_2	f_1	f_2
DK15-4	8	65	6	69
DK4-3	5	75	5	73
DC-4	6	70	7	66

6. Comparison of release profiles of different tablets prepared

Table: 20 Release kinetics of different optimized formulations

Formulation codes of best formulations	R^2 values								Release exponent (n)	
	Zero order		First order		Higuchi		Peppas			
	LD	CD	LD	CD	LD	CD	LD	CD	LD	CD
DK15-4	0.939	0.942	0.832	0.833	0.993	0.989	0.989	0.991	0.62	0.63
DK4-4	0.875	0.879	0.728	0.730	0.962	0.960	0.963	0.963	0.72	0.74
DC-4	0.922	0.925	0.853	0.851	0.994	0.993	0.996	0.995	0.58	0.59

Conclusion: Upon comparison of correlation co-efficient values (R^2) of all the best formulations from the different batches, it was indicated that the release profiles of Levodopa and Carbidopa are close to zero order and follow diffusion dependent release as the values are close to one.

5.7. STABILITY RESULTS OF THE BEST FORMULAE

Table: 21

Drug content in the tablets exposed to different stability conditions

Formulation code		Initial	2-8°C		25±2°C/60±5% RH		40±2°C/75±5% RH		Photo stability study	
			30 days	60 days	30 days	60 days	30 days	60 days	30 days	60 days
Levodopa	DK15-4	98.24	98.20	98.00	97.81	97.81	95.55	94.85	97.28	97.11
	DK4-3	97.98	97.9	97.85	97.01	97.28	94.74	94.16	96.39	96.15
	DC –4	97.41	97.32	97.19	98.03	96.96	94.47	94.13	96.82	96.46
Carbidopa	DK15-4	97.32	97.12	97.01	97.12	97.03	95.24	94.14	94.12	93.94
	DK4-3	99.76	98.97	98.36	97.28	97.18	96.75	96.24	94.27	94.03
	DC-4	99.56	98.95	98.89	97.74	97.67	95.44	95.11	92.87	92.14

REFERENCES

1. Chiao, C. S .L., Robinson, J.R., 1995. Sustained Release Drug Deliver Systems in Remington - The science and Practice of Pharmacy 19th Ed Mack Publishing Company.

2. Colombo, P., Bettini, R., Peppas, N. A., 1999. Observation of swelling process and diffusion front position during swelling in hydroxypropyl methylcellulose (HPMC) matrices containing a soluble drug. J. Contr. Rel. 61, 83-91.

3. Colombo, P., Bettini, R., Santi, P., De Ascentiis, A., Peppas, N. A., 1996. Analysis of the swelling and release mechanisms from drug delivery systems with emphasis on drug solubility and water transport. J. Contr. Rel. 39, 231- 237.

4. Colombo, P., Bettini, R., Santi, Peppas, N. A., 2001 Swellable matrices for controlled drug delivery: gel layer behavior, mechanisms and optimal performance, Pharm. Sci. Tech. Today 3, 198-204.

5. Dabbagh, M. A.; Ford, J. L., Rubenstein, M. H., Hogan, J. E., Rajabi- Siahboomi, A. R., 1999. Release of propranolol hydrochloride from matrix tablets containing sodium carboxymethylcellulose. Pharm. Dev.Tech. 4, 313- 324.

6. Dahl, T. C., Calderwood, T., Bormeth, A., Trimble, K. and Piepmeier, E., 1990 Influence of physio-chemical properties of hydroxypropyl methylcellulose on naproxen release from sustained-release matrix tablets. J. Controlled Release 14: 1-10.

7. Dow Pharmaceutical Excipients, 1996. Formulating for controlled release with Methocel Premium cellulose ethers. The Dow Chemical Company, Midland, Michigan.

8. Evaluation of the New Polyvinylacetate/Povidone Excipient for Matrix Sustained Release Dosage Forms, Pharm. Ind, 63, 624-629.

9. Eriksen, S., 1970 in The Theory and Practice of Industrial Pharmacy (L. Lachman, H. A. Lieberman, and J. L. Kanig, Lea & Febiger, Philadelphia, 408.

10. FDA, 1997. ICH Q1C Stability Testing for New Dosage Forms. Guidance for Industry. US Department of Health and Human Services Food and Drug Administration Center for Drug Evaluation and Research, Center for Biologics Evaluation and Research, ICH.

11. FDA, 1997a. Modified Release Solid Oral Dosage Forms. Scale-Up and Post approval Changes: Chemistry, Manufacturing, and Controls, *In Vitro* dissolution Testing and *In Vivo* Bioequivalence Documentation. Guidance for Industry. US Department of Health and Human Services Food and Drug Administration Center for Drug Evaluation and Research, Center for Biologics Evaluation and Research.

12. FDA, 1997b. Extended Release Solid Oral Dosage Forms Development, Evaluation and Application Of *In Vitro-In Vivo* Correlation. Guidance for Industry. US Department of Health and Human Services, Food and Drug Administration, Center for Drug Evaluation and Research.

13. FDA, 2001. ICH Q1A Stability Testing of New Drug Substances and Products Guidance for industry. US Department of Health and Human Services Food and Drug Administration Center for Drug Evaluation and Research, Center for Biologics Evaluation and Research, ICH.

14. FDA, 2001. Statistical Approaches to Establishing Bioequivalence. Guidance for Industry. US Department of Health and Human Services, Food and Drug Administration, Center for Drug Evaluation and Research.

15. Feely, L. C., Davis, S. S., 1988. Influence of polymeric excipients on drug release from hydroxypropylmethylcellulose matrices. Int. J. Pharm. 41, 83-90.

16. Ford, J. L., Rubinstein, M. H., Hogan, J. E., 1985. Dissolution of a poorly water soluble drug, indomethacin, from HPMC controlled release tablets. J. Pharm. Pharmacol. 37, 33.

17. Gao, P, Nixon, P. R, Skoug, J. W., 1995. Diffusion in HPMC gels II. Prediction of drug release rates from hydrophilic matrix extended-release dosage forms, Pharm Res. 12,965-971.

18. Higuchi, T., 1963. Mechanism of Sustained Action Medication: Theoretical Analysis of Rate of Release of Solid Drugs Dispersed in Solid Matrices. J. Pharm. Sci. 52, 1145-1149.

19. Hogan, J.E., 1989. Hydroxypropylmethylcellulose sustained release technology.Drug Dev. Ind. Pharm. 15, 975-999.

20. Jantzen, G. M., Robinson, J. R., 1996. Sustained- and Controlled-Release Drug Delivery Systems in Modern Pharmaceutics, 3rd Ed (Banker G., Rhodes, C. Edts). Marcel Dekker Inc.

21. Lee, V. H., Robinson, J. R., 1978 in Sustained and Controlled Release Drug Delivery Systems, J. R. Robinson, Marcel Dekker, New York, NY, 71-121.

22. Mitchell, K.; Ford, J. L.; Armstrong, D. J.; Elliott, P. N. C.; Hogan, J. E.,Rostron, C., 1993. The influence of drugs on the properties of gels and swelling characteristics of matrices containing methylcellulose and hydroxypropylmethyl cellulose. Int.J.Pharm. 100, 165-173.

23. Nellore, R. V., Rekhi, G. S., Hussain, A. S., Tillman, L. G., Augsburger, L. L., 1998. Development of metoprolol tartrate extended release matrix tablet formulations for regulatory policy consideration. J. Contr. Rel. 50, 247-256.

24. Peppas, N. A., 1985. Analysis of Fickian and Non-Fickian Drug Release from polymers. Pharm. Acta. Helv. 60, 110-111.

25. Peppas, N. A., Colombo, P., 1997. Analysis of drug release behavior from swellable polymer carriers using the dimensionality index. J. Contr. Rel. 45, 35.

26. Peppas, N. A., Sahlin, J. J., 1989. A simple equation for the description of solute release. III. Coupling of diffusion and relaxation. Int. J. Pharm. 57, 169-172.

27. Perez-Marcos, B., Ford, J. L., Armstrong, D. J., Elliot, P. N. C., Rostron, C., Hogan, J. E., 1994. Release of propranolol hydrochloride from matrix tablets containing hydroxypropylmethylcellulose K4M an carbopol 974. Int.J.Pharm. 111, 251-259.

28. PK Solutions 2.0™. Summit Research Services, Montrose CA. Plazier, V.J.; Dauwe, D., Brioen, P., 1997 S.T.P. Pharma Sci. 7(6) 491-497.

29. Po, A. L. W., Wong, L. P., Gilligan, C. A., 1990 Characterization of commercially available theophylline sustained release or controlled release systems in vitro drug release profiles Int.J.Pharm. 66, 111-130.

30. Qiu, Y., Zhang, G., 2000. Research and Development Aspects of Oral Controlled-Release Dosage Forms in Handbook of Pharmaceutical Controlled Release Technology (Wise, D. L. Edt), Marcel Dekker Inc.

31. Rajabi-Siahboomi, A. R., Jordan, M.P., 2000. Slow release HOMC matrix systems. Eur Pharm Rev. 5: 21-23.

32. Rekhi, G. S., Nellore, R. V., Hussain, A. S., Tillman, L. G., Augsburger, L. L., et al., 1999. Identification of critical formulation and processing variables for metoprolol tartrate extended-release (ER) matrix tablets. J. Contr. Rel. 59, 327-342.

33. Ritschel, W. A., 1992 Handbook of Basic Pharmacokinetics, Fourth Edition, Drug Intelligence Publications Inc., Hamilton, IL.,515-516.

34. Robinson, J. R., Lee, V. H. L., 1987 in Controlled Drug Delivery: Fundamentals and Applications, Second Edition, Marcel Dekker, Inc. New York, NY,372-373.

35. Shao, Z. J., Farooqi, M. I., Diaz, S., Krishna, A. K., Muhammad, N. A., 2001. Effects of formulation variables and postcompression curing on drug release from a new sustained release matrix material: polyvinylacetate povidone. Pharm. Dev. Techol. 6, 247-254.

36. Siepmann, J., Kranz, H., 2000. Calculation of the required size and shape of hydroxypropyl methylcellulose matrices to achieve desired drug release profiles. Int. J. Pharm. 200, 151-164

37. Siepmann, J., Kranz, H., Bodmeier, R., Peppas, N. A., 1999a. HPMC matrices for controlled drug delivery: new model combining diffusion, swelling, and dissolution mechanisms and predicting the release kinetics. Pharm. Res.16, 1748-1756.

38. Siepmann, J., Lecomte, F., Bodmeier, R., 1999b. Diffusion-controlled drug delivery systems: calculation of the required composition to achieve desired release profiles. J. Contr. Rel. 60, 379-389.

39. Siepmann, J., Podual, K., Sriwongjanya, M., Peppas, N. A., Bodmeier, R., 1999c. New model describing the swelling and drug release kinetics from hydroxypropyl methylcellulose tablets. J. Pharm. Sci. 88, 65-72.

40. Sung, K. C., Nixon, P. R., Skoug, J. W., Ju, T. R., Patel, M. V., et al., 1996. Effect of formulation variables on drug and polymer release from HPMC based matrix tablets. Int. J. Pharm. 142, 53-60.

41. Takka, S., Rajbhandari, S., Sakr, A., 2001. Effect of anionic polymers on the release of propranolol hydrochloride from matrix tablets. Eur. J. Pharm. Biopharm. 52, 75-82.

42. Tillotson, J., 2004. Development and evaluation of extended release bumetanide tablets. Ph.D. Dissertation, University of Cincinnati.

43. United States Pharmacopeia & National Formulary 26th Ed. The United States Pharmacopeial Convention Inc., 2003.

44. Upadrashta, S. M., Katikaneni, P. R., Hileman, G. A., Keshary, P. R., 1993. Direct compression controlled release tablets using ethylcellulose matrices. Drug Dev. Ind. Pharm. 19, 449-460.

45. Velasco, M. V., Ford, J. L., Rowe, P., Rajabi-Siahboomi, A. R., 1999. Influence of compression force on the release of diclofenac sodium from HPMC tablets. J. Contr. Rel. 57, 75-85.

46. Venkatraman, S., Davar, N., Chester, A., Kleiner, L., 2000. An Overview of Controlled-Release Systems in Handbook of Pharmaceutical Controlled Release Technology (Wise, D. L. Edt), Marcel Dekker Inc.

47. Wagner J. G., 1971. Biopharmaceutics and Relevant Pharmacokinetics, Drug Intelligence Publishers, Illinois.

48. Gwen M. Jantzen and Joseph R Robinson, Sustained and Controlled Release   drug delivery systems, In Modern pharmaceutics, Marcel Decker, 1996, Vol 72.3rd edition, 575.

49. Lordi N.G., Lachman L; Liberman H.A and Kanig J.L. The theory and practice of industrial pharmacy, Varghese publication house Bombay, third edition, 1987, 430-435.

50. Herbert A. Liberman, Leon Lachaman, Joseph B. Schwartz, Pharmaceutical Dosage forms – Tablets, 2nd edition. 274-279.

51. Brahmankar D.M., Jaiswal S.B. Biopharmaceutics and Pharmacokinetics. A Treatise, Reprint 2001, 335-357

52. Physicians Desk references 56th edition & 1030-1091, 2692-2696.

53. Gibson. M. Pharmaceutical Preformulation and formulation. A practical guide for   candidate drug selection to commercial dosage form, 2004, 379-458.

54. Indian Pharmacopoeia, Volume 11, 1996. Volume-1, 91-92.

55. British Pharmacopoeia- 1993, volume-1, 73.

56. The Merck index, An encyclopedia of chemicals, drugs& biologicals., Thirteenth edition-2001,1727

57. Analytical profiles of drug substances, volume-20

58. James E.F. Reynolds, Matrindale, The Extra Pharmacopoeia, 527.

59. S.J. Desai, A.P. Sonelli and W.I. Higuchi, 1965, Investigation factors influencing release of solid drug dispersed in inert matrices. J.pharm Sci., 54, 1145.

60. Alfonso R Gennaro, Controlled release drug delivery systems: The science and practice of pharmacy, Remington 20[th]Edition, vol.1, 903-930.

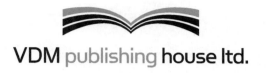

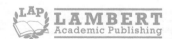
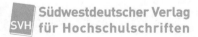

Made in United States
Troutdale, OR
03/05/2024

18242336R00046